Discovering Scandi Sense Diet

A Fresh Approach to Weight Management and Well-being

Donna Johnson

Copyright 2023-

Donna Johnson

ISBN

Printed in the United States of America

Disclaimer

Table of Contents

Introduction

Unveiling the Scandinavian Way to a Healthier You

Hi, guy, you're there finding a sustainable, rational, and really successful approach to healthy eating may be difficult and confusing in a world full of fad diets, weight reduction schemes, and contradicting nutritional advice. It's simple to get disoriented by the deluge of information and not know which direction to go in your pursuit of a better, livelier existence.

The Scandi Sense Diet is a novel approach to eating that combines the ideas of balance, diversity, and proportion into a nutritional tapestry that promises long-term health and a healthier, more energetic version of yourself. It is amazingly successful and refreshingly sensible. We cordially welcome you to go with us on a voyage of self-discovery as we unlock the Scandinavian keys to long-term health and balanced nutrition.

We start our adventure by revealing the Scandi Sense Diet, a Scandinavian eating philosophy that has been subtly altering people's lives and waistlines all around the globe. Discover the history and tenets of this dietary philosophy in these pages, and leave with a deep comprehension of why it endures and what makes it different from the other diets that have come and gone. The Scandi Sense Diet, which is often referred to as a way of life rather than a diet, places a strong emphasis on proportion, diversity, and balance as the keys to realizing your maximum health potential.

The Nordic Way of Eating

Scandinavia has always captivated our hearts with its stunning landscapes, breathtaking fjords, and energetic towns. But the Nordic nations are distinct for more reasons than simply their landscapes. They are also the center of a culinary culture that emphasizes balance, simplicity, and fresh, in-season ingredients. We'll look at the fundamentals of Nordic nutrition and how the Scandi Sense Diet is built upon them.

Why Scandi Sense Is Effective?

As they say, the evidence is in the pudding. We'll explore the science and studies that back up the effectiveness of the Scandi Sense Diet. You'll learn why it's a comprehensive, evidence-based strategy to controlling your weight, enhancing your health, and adopting a fulfilling and healthy lifestyle rather than simply another diet fad. This chapter will prepare you for the change you're about to experience.

Along the way, you will learn how to apply the concepts and methods of the Scandi Sense Diet to your everyday life in addition to learning about them. We'll walk you through the practice of portion management, meal planning, and mindful eating, assisting you in transforming these ideas into doable actions that promote a happier, healthier you.

It's time to embrace a more sustainable, fun, and well-balanced way of eating and bid adieu to the confusion and mayhem of contemporary diets. For anyone looking for a longer-term solution to live a better, more energetic life, the Scandi Sense Diet is an excellent choice. Are you prepared to start this life-changing adventure of learning about Scandi Sense? If yes, let's start the journey towards health together, one tasty and well-balanced meal at a time, by turning the page.

Chapter 1

Building Blocks of Scandi Sense

It's crucial to begin our exploration of Scandi Sense by comprehending the fundamental ideas that underpin the longevity and effectiveness of this Scandinavian eating philosophy. The foundation of this common sense and environmentally friendly approach to bodily nourishment is the "Building Blocks of Scandi Sense".

Proportion, Variety, and Balance

Three fundamental components make up the Scandi Sense Diet: proportion, variety, and balance. These ideas represent the cornerstone of how Scandinavians view eating, not merely some rules to follow.

1. Balance: The foundation of Scandi Sense is balance. It entails the skill of tastefully blending various dietary categories and nutrients. Rather of stigmatizing certain foods or banning whole food categories, the Scandi Sense Diet promotes moderation. The goal is to provide your body a wide range of nutrients by including a variety of carbs, proteins, fats, and veggies into your meals.

2. Variety: Another essential component of the Scandi Sense Diet is variety. A wide variety of

meals, in terms of ingredients and tastes, are celebrated in the Nordic diet. This diversity guarantees that you get a broad range of nutrients in addition to adding interest and enjoyment to your meals.

3. Proportion: The third pillar of Scandi Sense is proportion. It draws attention to the proportions of the various meals on your plate and the quantity of your servings. Understanding portion management and using the "Scandi Sense Plate" as a visual tool to help with meal planning are important components of the Scandi Sense methodology.

The Scandi Earbud

The Scandi Sense Plate is the central idea of the Scandi Sense Diet. It's a picture manual that will assist you in preparing wholesome, well-balanced meals. Each portion of the plate is designated for a different dietary category, such as vegetables, proteins, carbs, and fats. You may create balanced meals that adhere to the concepts of balance, variety, and proportion with ease by using this model.

1. Veggies: The biggest portion of the plate, veggies are high in fiber, vitamins, and minerals. This

encourages you to eat a lot of them. They provide vital nutrients and serve as the basis for your meals.

2. Proteins: A significant amount of the plate is made up of proteins, which may be found in fish, poultry, dairy, and plant-based foods. They are essential for immunological response, muscular healing, and general health.

3. Carbohydrates: Energy cannot be produced without carbohydrates. A section of the Scandi Sense Plate is dedicated to carbs, with an emphasis on nutritious grains and starches that maintain energy levels without spiking blood sugar.

4. Fats: There is a place on the plate for healthy fats, such those in nuts, seeds, and certain oils. These fat are critical for hormone synthesis, brain function, and general wellness.

Chapter 2

The Nordic Pantry

One of the keys to success in the quest for Discovering Scandi Sense is found in your kitchen, more precisely in your pantry. The Scandi Sense Diet is realized in the Nordic Pantry, which is filled with necessary items that represent the Nordic diet. We will examine the essential elements of the Nordic Pantry in this chapter, offering an understanding of the items that serve as the foundation for this sane and nutritious eating strategy.

Primitive Components for Nordic Sense Cooking

Nutrient-dense, natural foods that have undergone little processing are highly valued in The Nordic Pantry. The following are essential components of a fully supplied Scandi Sense kitchen:

1. Whole Grains: Oats, rye, barley, and whole wheat are among the entire grains that Scandinavians like. These grains should be a staple in your cupboard since they are high in fiber and provide you long-lasting energy.

2. Fish: A mainstay of the Nordic diet are fatty fish like salmon, mackerel, and herring. They are

great providers of heart- and brain-healthy omega-3 fatty acids.

3. Lean Proteins: Scandi Sense recipes often call for poultry, lean meat cuts, and lentils as protein sources. For the general health and well-being of muscles, several proteins are essential.

4. Dairy Products: Nordic kitchens often include low-fat dairy items like yogurt and milk. They provide vital elements for digestive health, including as probiotics and calcium.

5. Root Vegetables: Scandinavian cooking often uses root vegetables including potatoes, carrots, and turnips. They provide dietary fiber, vitamins, and minerals.

6. Berries: High in antioxidants, berries such as lingonberries, blues, and cloudberries are often used in classic Scandinavian jams and pastries.

7. Herbs and Spices: You may flavor food without using a lot of salt or fat by adding herbs like parsley and dill. Cardamom and cinnamon are two vital spices for baked goods.

8. Healthy Fats: A key component of the Scandi Sense Diet are healthy fats, which may be found in nuts, seeds, and specific oils like rapeseed and canola.

Known for their efficiency and simplicity, Scandinavian kitchens may be a source of inspiration for implementing the Scandi Sense Diet. Equipping your kitchen with Scandinavian essentials will not only facilitate meal preparation but also harmonize your kitchen with the three main tenets of this food philosophy: balance, diversity, and proportion. This is how you do it:

1. Give Whole Foods Priority: The Scandi Sense Diet is based on whole, minimally processed foods. When restocking your pantry, give special attention to lean proteins such as fish and chicken, nutritious grains like oats, barley, and rye, and an assortment of fruits and vegetables. Choose foods that are as near to their original condition as you can.

2. Tidy and Organize: Disarray and bad eating habits might result from a disorganized kitchen. Kitchens in the Scandinavian style are renowned for their order and simplicity. Organize your pantry, refrigerator, and cabinets to reduce clutter and get rid of superfluous goods. This will motivate you to cook more at home by making it easier for you to get ingredients.

3. Quality above Quantity: When it comes to food, Scandinavians value quality above quantity. Invest on long-lasting, premium food and utensils. This improves the taste of your food while lowering waste and encouraging a more environmentally friendly way of eating.

4. Seasoned and Local Produce: Adopt the Nordic custom of consuming locally grown and in season food. In addition to tasting better, in-season food is higher in nutrients. To lessen your carbon footprint, pick foods that are farmed nearby and support your local farmers and markets.

5. Mindful Shopping: Approach your shopping with awareness. Before you go shopping, make a list to help you resist impulsive buys. To make educated decisions and know what you're purchasing, read the food labels. Choose foods that have less artificial chemicals, preservatives, and additives.

6. Adopt simple equipment: In terms of appliances and equipment, Scandinavian kitchens are often simple. Invest in a few high-quality, multipurpose utensils that may be used for several tasks. This promotes inventive and innovative cooking in addition to clearing clutter.

7. Minimize Food Waste: People from Scandinavia are famed for their attempts to cut down on food waste. Make a plan for your meals, think of inventive ways to utilize leftovers, and use foods that could otherwise go bad. Another ecological habit to think about is composting.

8. Sustainable Packaging: Select goods that come in environmentally friendly packaging to lessen your impact on the environment. Avoid using single-use plastics as much as possible and look for reusable or recyclable containers.

9. Incorporate Nordic Flavors: To give your meals a Nordic flavor, try experimenting with herbs and spices from Scandinavia. A few examples include cinnamon, cardamom, and dill. Not only can these tastes improve your food, they also improve your health in general.

Shopping Tips and Tricks

Making deliberate grocery store selections is crucial to following the Scandi Sense Diet to the fullest. Your buying habits should reflect the simple and orderly style that characterizes Scandinavian kitchens. To assist you in embracing the Scandi Sense approach to food buying, consider the following shopping tips and tricks:

1. Plan Your Meals and Make a List: Spend some time organizing your weekly menu before you go shopping. Make a shopping list that includes the foods you'll need depending on your meal plan. This will assist you in avoiding rash purchases and maintaining focus on your nutritional objectives.

2. Adhere to the Perimeter: Upon entering a grocery shop, you'll see that the fresh and complete goods, such as meats, dairy products, and vegetables, are often found along the store's perimeter. These are the mainstays of the Diet Scandi Sense. This is where you should spend most of your time while shopping; avoid the middle aisles, which are often filled with processed and unhealthy goods.

3. Examine Food Labels: Give food labels a thorough reading and comprehension. Seek for goods with the fewest artificial substances, preservatives, and additives possible. Verify that the goods adhere to the principles of balance, diversity, and proportion by looking at the nutrition information. Pay close attention to serving quantities and additional sugars.

4. Pick entire Grains: Give entire grains like oats, barley, and whole wheat priority when choosing grains. These grains are high in vital minerals and fiber. Instead of refined rice, pasta, and bread, choose whole-grain options.

5. Shop locally and seasonally: Adopt the Scandinavian eating custom of purchasing locally and seasonally. Seasonally available vegetables is frequently more tasty and nutrient-dense. Assist regional farmers and markets to lessen your effect on the environment and improve your ties to the neighborhood.

6. Purchase Both Fresh and Frozen Produce: While fresh produce is excellent, frozen alternatives are just as wholesome and practical. To guarantee you have access to wholesome foods at all times, stock your freezer with a selection of frozen fruits and veggies.

7. Increase Your Lean Protein Intake: Pick lean protein sources like tofu, skinless chicken, fish, and lentils. These choices are low in saturated fat and high in protein. Think about making bulk purchases and freezing excess portions for later use.

8. Reduce Processed Foods: Purchase as little processed and highly packaged foods as possible. These often have artificial ingredients, harmful fats, and hidden sugars. When you go grocery shopping, make fresh, healthy foods your main focus.

9. Be Aware of Portion amounts: When purchasing packaged goods, pay attention to the portion amounts. Proportion is important while following the Scandi Sense Diet, so think about how the product's size fits into your overall nutritional objectives.

10. Take into Account Sustainable Packaging: Whenever feasible, choose items with environmentally friendly packaging. Try to utilize reusable or recyclable containers instead of single-use plastics. One tiny but effective method to support companies who are devoted to sustainability is to support brands that share this commitment.

11. Steer Clear of Shopping While Hungry: Making impulsive, unhealthy food selections while shopping on an empty stomach might lead to poor decisions. Before you go to the market, have a

little lunch or snack to help you stay on your shopping list and make wiser choices.

Chapter 3

Mindful Eating the Scandi Way

One of the main components of the Scandi Sense Diet is mindful eating. It matters how you eat as much as what you consume. This chapter will examine the idea of mindful eating in a Scandi context and discuss the significant effects it may have on both your relationship with food and your general state of health.

The Art of Savoring

Part of the core of the Scandi Sense Diet is to savor your meal. Eating in the Scandinavian style encourages you to take your time and savor your food. Rather of hurrying through your meal, supper, or breakfast, savor each mouthful and its colors, textures, and tastes. You'll discover that, if you taste your meal, smaller servings may be just as fulfilling as bigger ones. Gaining increased awareness of your body's hunger and fullness cues helps you quit eating when you're content rather than stuffed.

Slowing Down and Savoring Each Bite

Slowing down the speed of your meals is one of the keys to mindful eating. It's simple to eat quickly in our fast-paced society when you're preoccupied with devices, work, or other commitments. The Scandi approach advocates for uninterrupted mealtimes that are devoted to mealtimes. Make sure that your dining area is calm and concentrated by turning off the TV and putting your phone away. This enables you to thoroughly appreciate and pay attention to your meal.

Savor the flavor, texture, and scent with every mouthful. Thank you for the sustenance and the work that went into making your lunch. By doing this, you may avoid overeating and improve your pleasure of food by learning to identify when you're full.

Eating with All Your Senses

When dining in the Scandi style, every sensation is involved. Aspects such as touch, scent, sight, and even sound influence your experience. For instance:

- Sight: Pause to appreciate the hues and arrangement of your dish. A vibrant meal full of different veggies may be inviting and visually pleasing.
- Smell: Your hunger might be strongly stimulated by the smell of your meal. Take a deep breath and enjoy the aromas rising from your dish.

- Touch: Take note of the food's textures. Is it soft, creamy, or crispy? Examining the textures and flavors of your food may be enjoyable.

- Sound: The noises associated with preparing and eating, like the crunch of fresh vegetables or the sizzle of a frying pan, enhance the sensory richness of your meal.

Chapter 4

Portion Control and Proportion

Portion management and proportion are essential ideas in the realm of the Scandi Sense Diet that direct your eating patterns. In order to help you develop a sustainable and balanced eating plan, this chapter delves into the significance of comprehending and putting into practice portion management and proportion.

Avoiding Overindulgence

You may prevent overindulgence by using portion control and proportion, which is one of their major advantages. Unknowingly consuming large quantities might result in weight gain and other health problems for a lot of individuals. You may make better decisions and become more aware of how much food you consume by using the Scandi Sense Plate as a guide.

Understanding Portion Sizes

Understanding meal portions and energy composition is important according to the Scandi Sense Diet. This information gives you the ability to plan meals and regulate portions with understanding. The diet encourages you to estimate portion sizes by using visual clues rather than exact calorie counting or weighing.

You may have a more positive connection with food by learning to use the Scandi Sense Plate to determine portion sizes and paying attention to your body's signals of hunger and fullness. You'll discover that you may enjoy your meals without feeling deprived or overindulging if you eat in moderation and manage your servings.

An easy and efficient method to get a balanced and wholesome diet is to include the Scandi Sense Diet's recommendations for portion management and proportion into your eating habits. It encourages a more conscious way of eating, which enables you to enjoy your food and take better care of your weight and general health.

Chapter 5

Meal Planning and Preparation

Weekly Meal Plan

The Scandi Sense Diet focuses on mindful portion control and balanced meals.

Here's a comprehensive 7-day meal plan with Scandi Sense Diet principles in mind:

Day 1:

Breakfast: Scandi Sense Oatmeal

Ingredients:

- 40g whole-grain oats
- 150g plain Greek yogurt
- Sliced banana or berries (optional)
- A drizzle of honey or maple syrup (optional)

Instructions:

1. Gather Your Ingredients: Collect all the necessary ingredients, including whole-grain oats, plain Greek yogurt, and any optional toppings like sliced banana, berries, honey, or maple syrup.

2. Measure the Oats: Measure out 40g of whole-grain oats. You can adjust the quantity to suit your preference or dietary needs.

3. Combine Oats and Greek Yogurt: In a bowl, mix the measured whole-grain oats with 150g of plain Greek yogurt. The yogurt adds creaminess and protein to the oatmeal.

4. Stir Well: Stir the oats and yogurt together until they are well combined. You can adjust the thickness of the oatmeal by adding more or less yogurt.

5. Add Toppings (Optional): If desired, add sliced banana, berries, or other toppings to your oatmeal. These can add sweetness and extra flavor.

6. Drizzle with Honey or Maple Syrup (Optional): If you prefer a sweeter oatmeal, you can drizzle a small amount of honey or maple syrup over the top. Remember to use these sweeteners in moderation to align with the Scandi Sense Diet principles.

7. Serve: Your Scandi Sense Oatmeal is ready to be enjoyed. Serve it immediately for a fresh and satisfying breakfast.

The preparation time for Scandi Sense Oatmeal is minimal, typically taking around 5 minutes or less. It's a quick and easy breakfast option that you can put together in the morning or even prepare the night before and store in the refrigerator for a grab-and-go meal. The duration may vary depending on how quickly you can measure and mix the ingredients and whether you choose to add optional toppings or sweeteners.

Lunch: Scandi Sense Smørrebrød

Ingredients:

- Whole-grain rye bread slices
- Lean protein (e.g., turkey or chicken)
- Sliced tomatoes
- Sliced cucumbers
- Greek yogurt or a light mayo-based dressing
- Fresh dill or other herbs for garnish

Instructions:

1. Gather your Ingredients: Collect whole-grain rye bread, lean protein of your choice (turkey or chicken), sliced tomatoes, sliced cucumbers, Greek yogurt or a light mayo-based dressing, and fresh dill or other herbs for garnish.

2. Prep the Bread: Take one or two slices of whole-grain rye bread for each sandwich. Rye bread is a traditional choice, but you can use any whole-grain bread that aligns with your dietary preferences.

3. Spread a Light Dressing: Spread a thin layer of Greek yogurt or a light mayo-based dressing on the bread slices. This serves as a base and adds moisture to the sandwich.

4. Add Lean Protein: Place a generous portion (about 100g) of lean protein (turkey or chicken) on top of the dressing.

5. Layer with Vegetables: Add a layer of sliced tomatoes and cucumbers on top of the protein. You can also add other vegetables like lettuce or bell peppers for extra freshness and flavor.

6. Garnish: Finish your Smørrebrød with fresh dill or other herbs for garnish. Fresh herbs add a delightful Scandinavian touch.

7. Serve: Your Scandi Sense Smørrebrød is ready to be served. These open-faced sandwiches are perfect for a light lunch or snack.

The preparation time for Scandi Sense Smørrebrød is minimal, usually taking around 5-10 minutes. The key to this dish is the assembly of fresh ingredients. You can adjust the number of sandwiches you make to fit your needs. It's a convenient and healthy meal option that you can prepare quickly and enjoy in no time.

Dinner: Scandi Sense Baked Salmon

Ingredients:

- Salmon fillets
- Fresh dill
- Lemon slices
- Olive oil
- Salt and pepper to taste

Instructions:

1. Preheat the Oven: Preheat your oven to 375°F (190°C). This is the standard temperature for baking salmon.
2. Prepare the Salmon: Place the salmon fillets on a baking sheet lined with parchment paper or in a baking dish. Make sure the salmon fillets are skin-side down for even cooking.
3. Season the Salmon: Drizzle a bit of olive oil over the salmon to prevent it from sticking to the baking

sheet or dish. Season the salmon with salt and pepper to taste.

4. Add Fresh Dill and Lemon: Sprinkle fresh dill over the salmon fillets. You can use as much or as little dill as you prefer. Lay lemon slices over the salmon for added flavor.

5. Bake the Salmon: Place the baking sheet or dish in the preheated oven. Bake the salmon for about 12-15 minutes per inch of thickness. The salmon is done when it flakes easily with a fork. Keep in mind that the exact cooking time may vary depending on the thickness of your salmon fillets.

6. Check for Doneness: To ensure the salmon is cooked to your liking, check its internal temperature with a meat thermometer. Salmon is safe to eat when it reaches 145°F (63°C).

7. Serve: Once the salmon is cooked to your satisfaction, remove it from the oven. Carefully transfer the salmon to serving plates.

The estimated preparation and cooking time for Scandi Sense Baked Salmon is around 20-25 minutes, depending on the thickness of your salmon fillets and your desired level of doneness. Keep in mind that this is a relatively quick and straightforward recipe, making it a convenient and healthy choice for a Scandi Sense meal.

Day 2:

Breakfast: Scandi Sense Cottage Cheese Parfait

Ingredients:

- 150g low-fat cottage cheese
- Fresh mixed berries (e.g., strawberries, blueberries, raspberries)
- A sprinkle of chopped nuts and seeds (e.g., almonds, walnuts, chia seeds)
- A drizzle of honey or maple syrup (optional)

Instructions:

1. Gather Your Ingredients: Collect low-fat cottage cheese, fresh mixed berries, chopped nuts and seeds, and honey or maple syrup (if using).
2. Layer the Cottage Cheese: Start by placing a layer of low-fat cottage cheese in a glass or a bowl. You can use a clear glass to create a visually appealing parfait.

3. Add Berries: Add a generous serving of fresh mixed berries on top of the cottage cheese. You can mix and match various berries for a burst of color and flavor.

4. Sprinkle Nuts and Seeds: Sprinkle a variety of chopped nuts and seeds over the berries and cottage cheese. This not only adds a satisfying crunch but also provides healthy fats and additional nutrients.

5. Drizzle with Honey or Maple Syrup (Optional): If you desire extra sweetness, you can drizzle a small amount of honey or maple syrup over the top of the parfait. Remember to use sweeteners sparingly to align with Scandi Sense Diet principles.

6. Repeat the Layers: If you're using a clear glass, you can create multiple layers by repeating the steps, alternating between cottage cheese, berries, nuts, and seeds.

7. Serve: Your Scandi Sense Cottage Cheese Parfait is ready to be served. Enjoy it as a healthy and delicious breakfast, snack, or dessert.

The preparation time for a Scandi Sense Cottage Cheese Parfait is minimal and should take approximately 5-10 minutes. The duration may vary depending on the time it takes to gather and chop the ingredients. This parfait is a quick and nutritious option for a satisfying and balanced meal.

Lunch: Scandi Sense Salad

Ingredients:

- A base of mixed greens (e.g., spinach, lettuce, arugula)
- Lean protein (e.g., grilled chicken, tofu, smoked salmon)
- Sliced cucumbers
- Cherry tomatoes
- Sliced bell peppers
- A simple dressing (olive oil and balsamic vinegar)
- Whole-grain rye crackers or bread (optional)

Instructions:

1. Gather your Ingredients: Collect the mixed greens, lean protein, cucumbers, cherry tomatoes, bell peppers, and dressing. Additionally, you can include whole-grain rye crackers or bread if desired.

2. Prepare the Greens: Wash and dry the mixed greens, then arrange them on a serving plate or in a salad bowl.

3. Add Lean Protein: Place a generous portion (about 100g) of lean protein (grilled chicken, tofu, and smoked salmon) on top of the mixed greens. This serves as the protein source for your salad.

4. Layer with Vegetables: Add sliced cucumbers, cherry tomatoes, and sliced bell peppers on top of the protein. Feel free to use other vegetables of your choice for added variety and freshness.

5. Dress the Salad: Drizzle the salad with a simple dressing made from olive oil and balsamic vinegar. You can adjust the dressing quantity to suit your preference.

6. Add Whole-Grain Rye Crackers or Bread (Optional): If you'd like to add whole-grain rye crackers or bread to your salad, you can serve them on the side.

7. Toss or Serve: If you prefer, you can gently toss the salad to mix the ingredients. Alternatively, serve it as a composed salad with distinct layers.

8. Serve: Your Scandi Sense Salad is ready to be served. Enjoy it as a satisfying and balanced meal.

The preparation time for a Scandi Sense Salad is quick and should take approximately 10-15 minutes, depending on how long it takes to wash and chop the ingredients and assemble the salad. The duration may vary based on your familiarity with the process and the number of ingredients you choose to include. This salad is an ideal choice for a healthy and refreshing meal.

Dinner: Scandi Sense Meatball Stew

Ingredients:

For the Meatballs:

- Lean ground meat (e.g., turkey or chicken)
- Breadcrumbs
- Chopped onion
- Egg (for binding)
- Salt and pepper
- Fresh herbs (e.g., parsley, dill)

For the Stew:

- Chicken or vegetable broth
- Carrots, peeled and chopped
- Celery, chopped
- Chopped tomatoes or tomato sauce

- Seasonings (e.g., bay leaves, thyme, salt, and pepper)

Instructions:

Meatball Preparation:

1. Mix the Meatball Ingredients: In a mixing bowl, combine the lean ground meat, breadcrumbs, chopped onion, egg, salt, pepper, and fresh herbs (such as parsley or dill). Mix until all the ingredients are well combined.
2. Form Meatballs: Shape the mixture into meatballs of your desired size. The size of the meatballs can vary based on your preference, but keep in mind that smaller meatballs will cook faster.

Stew Preparation:

3. Start the Stew: In a large pot, bring the chicken or vegetable broth to a simmer.
4. Add Vegetables: Add the chopped carrots and celery to the simmering broth. These vegetables will add flavor and nutrients to the stew.
5. Season the Stew: Season the stew with bay leaves, thyme, and salt and pepper to taste. Stir to combine.

6. Add the Meatballs: Gently add the meatballs to the simmering stew. Ensure they are submerged in the broth.

7. Simmer: Let the stew simmer for about 20-25 minutes, or until the meatballs are cooked through and the vegetables are tender.

8. Add Tomatoes (or Tomato Sauce): If desired, add chopped tomatoes or tomato sauce to the stew to create a flavorful base. Simmer for an additional 5-10 minutes.

9. Taste and Adjust: Taste the stew and adjust the seasoning if needed. You can add more salt, pepper, or herbs to suit your taste.

10. Serve: Your Scandi Sense Meatball Stew is ready to be served. Ladle the stew into bowls and enjoy.

The preparation and cooking time for Scandi Sense Meatball Stew typically takes around 45-60 minutes. This duration may vary based on factors like the size of the meatballs and the tenderness of the vegetables. It's a hearty and comforting dish that's worth the time it takes to prepare.

Day 3:

Breakfast: Scandi Sense Smoothie

Ingredients:

- 150g plain Greek yogurt
- A handful of spinach or other leafy greens
- 1 ripe banana
- A scoop of protein powder (optional)
- Water or milk for blending (e.g., almond milk or skim milk)

Instructions:

1. Gather Your Ingredients: Collect plain Greek yogurt, a handful of spinach or other leafy greens, a ripe banana, protein powder (if using), and your choice of liquid (water or milk).
2. Add Greek Yogurt: Place 150g of plain Greek yogurt in a blender. Greek yogurt provides protein and creaminess to the smoothie.
3. Add Leafy Greens: Add a handful of spinach or other leafy greens to the blender. This adds a boost of vitamins and fiber to your smoothie.
4. Add Banana: Peel the ripe banana and add it to the blender. The banana adds natural sweetness and creaminess to the smoothie.

5. Include Protein Powder (Optional): If you prefer extra protein, you can add a scoop of protein powder to the blender.

6. Pour in Liquid: Pour in your choice of liquid, whether it's water or milk, to facilitate blending. Start with a small amount and add more as needed to achieve your preferred smoothie consistency.

7. Blend: Blend all the ingredients until smooth and well combined. The blending duration may vary depending on your blender, but it typically takes around 1-2 minutes.

8. Taste and Adjust: Taste the smoothie and adjust the thickness or sweetness by adding more liquid or a touch of honey if desired.

9. Serve: Your Scandi Sense Smoothie is ready to be served. Pour it into a glass and enjoy it as a quick and nutritious breakfast or snack.

The preparation time for a Scandi Sense Smoothie is quick, usually taking around 5-10 minutes.

Lunch: Scandi Sense Tuna Salad

Ingredients:

- Canned tuna (in water or brine)

- Chopped red onion
- Chopped celery
- Light dressing (e.g., olive oil and lemon juice)
- Salt and pepper to taste
- Mixed greens (e.g., lettuce or spinach)

Instructions:

1. Gather Your Ingredients: Collect canned tuna, chopped red onion, chopped celery, a light dressing (such as a simple olive oil and lemon juice dressing), salt, pepper, and mixed greens.
2. Prepare the Tuna: Drain the canned tuna and transfer it to a mixing bowl.
3. Add Chopped Vegetables: Add the chopped red onion and celery to the tuna in the mixing bowl. These vegetables will provide texture and flavor to the salad.
4. Season the Salad: Season the mixture with salt and pepper to taste. Start with a small amount and adjust as needed.
5. Dress the Salad: Drizzle the salad with a light dressing. A simple combination of olive oil and lemon juice works well, but you can use your preferred dressing. The amount of dressing can be adjusted to your taste.

6. Mix: Gently mix the tuna, vegetables, and dressing until everything is well combined.

7. Serve on Mixed Greens: Place a bed of mixed greens (e.g., lettuce or spinach) on a serving plate or in a salad bowl. Top the greens with the tuna salad mixture.

8. Taste and Adjust: Taste the salad and adjust the seasoning or dressing if needed.

9. Serve: Your Scandi Sense Tuna Salad is ready to be served. Enjoy it as a quick and balanced meal for lunch or a light dinner.

The preparation time for a Scandi Sense Tuna Salad is minimal, taking approximately 10-15 minutes.

Dinner: Scandi Sense Veggie Stir-fry

Ingredients:

- Lean protein (e.g., chicken, tofu, or shrimp)
- Assorted vegetables (e.g., bell peppers, broccoli, carrots, snap peas)
- Olive oil or cooking oil of your choice
- Garlic and ginger (minced)
- Low-sodium soy sauce or a light stir-fry sauce
- Cooked whole grains (e.g., quinoa or brown rice)

Instructions:

1. Gather Your Ingredients: Collect your choice of lean protein (chicken, tofu, or shrimp), a variety of fresh vegetables (bell peppers, broccoli, carrots, snap peas, or your favorites), olive oil or cooking oil, minced garlic and ginger, low-sodium soy sauce or a light stir-fry sauce, and cooked whole grains (quinoa or brown rice).

2. Prepare the Protein: If you're using chicken or tofu, slice it into small, bite-sized pieces. If using shrimp, make sure they are peeled and deveined.

3. Cut the Vegetables: Chop the assorted vegetables into uniform, bite-sized pieces. Keep them separate from the protein.

4. Heat the Pan: Heat a large skillet or wok over medium-high heat. Add a small amount of olive oil or cooking oil.

5. Sauté Protein: Add the protein (chicken, tofu, or shrimp) to the hot skillet and cook until it's no longer pink (for chicken or tofu) or until the shrimp turn pink. Remove the cooked protein from the skillet and set it aside.

6. Sauté Garlic and Ginger: In the same skillet, add a bit more oil if needed. Sauté minced garlic and ginger for a minute or until fragrant.

7. Stir-Fry Vegetables: Add the chopped vegetables to the skillet and stir-fry for a few minutes until they start to become tender yet still crisp.

8. Combine Protein and Sauce: Return the cooked protein to the skillet and add low-sodium soy sauce or your preferred stir-fry sauce. Toss everything together and cook for a few more minutes until heated through and well coated with the sauce.

9. Serve Over Whole Grains: Place a serving of cooked whole grains (quinoa or brown rice) on a plate or in a bowl. Top the whole grains with the veggie and protein stir-fry.

10. Taste and Adjust: Taste the stir-fry and adjust the seasoning with additional sauce or soy sauce if desired.

The preparation and cooking time for a Scandi Sense Veggie Stir-Fry typically takes around 20-30 minutes.

Day 4:

Breakfast: Scandi Sense Porridge

Ingredients:

- 40g whole-grain oats
- Water or milk (e.g., skim milk, almond milk)
- Toppings of your choice (e.g., sliced strawberries, a dollop of yogurt, or a sprinkle of chopped nuts)

Instructions:

1. Gather Your Ingredients: Collect whole-grain oats, your choice of liquid (water or milk), and your preferred toppings.
2. Measure the Oats: Measure out 40g of whole-grain oats. Adjust the quantity to suit your preferences or dietary needs.
3. Add Liquid: In a saucepan, combine the measured oats with your choice of liquid (water or milk). The amount of liquid can vary based on how thick or thin you want your porridge. Typically, a 1:2 ratio of oats to liquid is a good starting point. You can adjust the ratio to achieve your desired consistency.
4. Heat the Mixture: Place the saucepan over medium heat and bring the oats and liquid to a gentle simmer.

5. Stir: Continuously stir the mixture as it cooks to prevent sticking and clumping. Stirring also helps to achieve a creamy consistency.

6. Cook: Allow the porridge to cook for about 5-10 minutes, or until it reaches your preferred thickness. If it gets too thick, you can add more liquid to reach your desired consistency.

7. Serve: Once the porridge is cooked to your liking, transfer it to a bowl.

8. Add Toppings: Top your Scandi Sense Porridge with your favorite toppings, such as sliced strawberries, a dollop of yogurt, or a sprinkle of chopped nuts.

9. Taste and Adjust: Taste the porridge and adjust the sweetness and thickness by adding more toppings or a drizzle of honey or maple syrup if desired.

10. Serve: Your Scandi Sense Porridge is ready to be served. Enjoy it as a comforting and balanced breakfast.

The preparation time for Scandi Sense Porridge is relatively short, taking around 10-15 minutes.

Lunch: Scandi Sense Wrap

Ingredients:

- Whole-grain wrap (e.g., whole-wheat tortilla or flatbread)
- Lean protein (e.g., grilled chicken, turkey, or tofu)
- Mixed greens (e.g., lettuce, spinach)
- Sliced vegetables (e.g., cucumber, bell pepper, tomato)
- Light dressing (e.g., olive oil and balsamic vinegar)
- Optional toppings (e.g., light mayo or mustard)

Instructions:

1. Gather Your Ingredients: Collect a whole-grain wrap, your choice of lean protein, mixed greens, sliced vegetables, a light dressing (such as a simple olive oil and balsamic vinegar dressing), and any optional toppings you prefer.
2. Prep the Wrap: Lay out the whole-grain wrap on a clean surface, such as a plate or a piece of parchment paper.
3. Add Lean Protein: Place a generous portion (about 100g) of your choice of lean protein (grilled chicken, turkey, or tofu) in the center of the wrap.

4. Layer with Vegetables: Add a layer of mixed greens, followed by sliced vegetables (e.g., cucumber, bell pepper, and tomato) on top of the protein. Feel free to include other vegetables to suit your taste.

5. Drizzle with Dressing: Drizzle the wrap with a light dressing made from olive oil and balsamic vinegar or your preferred dressing. This adds flavor and moisture to the wrap.

6. Add Optional Toppings: If you like, you can add optional toppings like a light mayo or mustard for extra flavor. Use these toppings in moderation to align with Scandi Sense Diet principles.

7. Wrap it Up: Fold the sides of the wrap over the filling, then roll it up from the bottom, creating a neat and compact wrap.

8. Taste and Adjust: Taste the wrap and adjust the seasoning or dressing if needed.

9. Serve: Your Scandi Sense Wrap is ready to be served. Enjoy it as a balanced and portable meal.

The preparation time for a Scandi Sense Wrap is minimal, typically taking around 10-15 minutes.

Dinner: Scandi Sense Baked Cod

Ingredients:

- Cod fillets
- Fresh dill
- Lemon slices
- Olive oil
- Salt and pepper to taste

Instructions:

1. Preheat the Oven: Preheat your oven to 375°F (190°C). This is the standard temperature for baking fish.
2. Prepare the Cod Fillets: Place the cod fillets on a baking sheet lined with parchment paper or in a baking dish. If the cod fillets have skin, make sure they are skin-side down.
3. Season the Cod: Drizzle a bit of olive oil over the cod fillets to prevent sticking and add moisture. Season the cod with salt and pepper to taste.
4. Add Fresh Dill and Lemon: Sprinkle fresh dill over the cod fillets. You can use as much or as little dill as you prefer. Lay lemon slices over the cod to add a burst of citrus flavor.
5. Bake the Cod: Place the baking sheet or dish in the preheated oven. Bake the cod for about 15-20

minutes, or until the fish is opaque and flakes easily with a fork. The exact cooking time may vary depending on the thickness of your cod fillets.

6. Check for Doneness: To ensure the cod is cooked to your liking, check its internal temperature with a meat thermometer. Cod is safe to eat when it reaches 145°F (63°C).

7. Serve: Once the cod is cooked to your satisfaction, remove it from the oven.

The preparation and cooking time for Scandi Sense Baked Cod typically takes around 20-25 minutes.

Day 5:

Breakfast: Scandi Sense Greek Yogurt Parfait

Ingredients:

- 150g plain Greek yogurt
- Fresh mixed berries (e.g., strawberries, blueberries, raspberries)
- A sprinkle of chopped nuts and seeds (e.g., almonds, walnuts, chia seeds)

Instructions:

1. Gather Your Ingredients: Collect plain Greek yogurt, fresh mixed berries, and chopped nuts and seeds.

2. Layer the Yogurt: Start by placing a layer of plain Greek yogurt in a glass or a bowl. You can use a clear glass to create an attractive parfait presentation.

3. Add Berries: Add a generous serving of fresh mixed berries on top of the Greek yogurt. You can mix and match various berries for a burst of color and flavor.

4. Sprinkle Nuts and Seeds: Sprinkle a variety of chopped nuts and seeds over the berries and yogurt. This not only adds a satisfying crunch but also provides healthy fats and additional nutrients.

5. Taste and Adjust: Taste the parfait and adjust the sweetness and thickness by adding more toppings or a drizzle of honey or maple syrup if desired.

6. Serve: Your Scandi Sense Greek Yogurt Parfait is ready to be served. Enjoy it as a healthy and delicious breakfast or snack.

The preparation time for a Scandi Sense Greek Yogurt Parfait is minimal and should take approximately 5-10 minutes.

Lunch: Scandi Sense Soup

Ingredients:

- Lean protein (e.g., chicken, turkey, tofu)
- Chopped vegetables (e.g., carrots, celery, onions)
- Low-sodium broth (e.g., chicken or vegetable)
- Seasonings (e.g., herbs, salt, pepper)
- Whole grains (e.g., barley, quinoa, or whole-wheat pasta)

Instructions:

1. Gather Your Ingredients: Collect your choice of lean protein (chicken, turkey, tofu), chopped vegetables, low-sodium broth, seasonings, and whole grains.
2. Prepare the Protein: If you're using chicken or tofu, slice it into small, bite-sized pieces.
3. Sauté Vegetables: In a large pot, heat a bit of olive oil or cooking oil over medium heat. Sauté the

chopped vegetables until they start to soften and become fragrant.

4. Add Protein: If you're using lean protein (chicken or tofu), add it to the pot and cook until it's no longer pink (for chicken) or until the tofu is heated through.

5. Add Broth: Pour in the low-sodium broth of your choice. The amount of broth can vary based on your preference and the consistency you desire for your soup. Typically, you'll need enough to cover the ingredients in the pot.

6. Season the Soup: Season the soup with your choice of herbs, salt, and pepper. This adds flavor to the soup. You can use seasonings like thyme, basil, or oregano for a Scandi-inspired touch.

7. Add Whole Grains: Include whole grains, such as barley, quinoa, or whole-wheat pasta, to the soup. These grains will provide heartiness and additional nutrients. Follow the package instructions for cooking times.

8. Simmer: Let the soup simmer for about 15-20 minutes, or until the vegetables and grains are tender and the flavors meld together.

9. Taste and Adjust: Taste the soup and adjust the seasoning if needed by adding more herbs, salt, or pepper.

10. Serve: Your Scandi Sense Soup is ready to be served. Ladle it into bowls and enjoy it as a comforting and balanced meal.

The preparation and cooking time for a Scandi Sense Soup typically takes around 30-40 minutes.

Dinner: Scandi Sense Grilled Turkey or Chicken

Ingredients:

- Turkey or chicken breast or thigh fillets
- Olive oil or a light marinade
- Salt and pepper to taste
- Optional herbs and spices for seasoning

Instructions:

1. Gather your Ingredients: Collect the turkey or chicken fillets, olive oil or a light marinade, salt, pepper, and any optional herbs and spices you'd like to use for seasoning.

2. Prep the Turkey or Chicken: If using whole turkey or chicken fillets, trim any excess fat. If the fillets

are thick, consider slicing them in half horizontally to ensure even cooking.

3. Season the Meat: Drizzle olive oil or a light marinade over the turkey or chicken fillets. Season with salt, pepper, and any additional herbs or spices. Rub the seasonings into the meat to ensure even distribution.

4. Preheat the Grill: Preheat your grill to medium-high heat. Make sure it's clean and well-oiled to prevent sticking.

5. Grill the Meat: Place the seasoned turkey or chicken fillets on the grill. Grill for approximately 6-8 minutes per side for chicken and 10-12 minutes per side for turkey, or until the meat is cooked through and has grill marks. The exact cooking time may vary depending on the thickness of the fillets and the heat of your grill.

6. Check for Doneness: To ensure the meat is fully cooked, use a meat thermometer to check its internal temperature. Chicken should reach 165°F (74°C), while turkey should reach 165°F (74°C) as well.

7. Rest the Meat: Remove the turkey or chicken from the grill and let it rest for a few minutes. This

allows the juices to redistribute, ensuring the meat remains tender and juicy.

8. Slice and Serve: Slice the grilled turkey or chicken fillets into serving portions. You can serve them with your choice of side dishes or salads.

The total preparation and grilling time for Scandi Sense Grilled Turkey or Chicken typically takes around 20-30 minutes.

Day 6:

Breakfast: Scandi Sense Breakfast Bowl

Ingredients:

- Greek yogurt or skyr
- Fresh mixed berries (e.g., strawberries, blueberries, raspberries)
- A sprinkle of chopped nuts and seeds (e.g., almonds, walnuts, chia seeds)
- A drizzle of honey or maple syrup (optional)
- Whole-grain muesli or granola (optional)

Instructions:

1. Gather Your Ingredients: Collect Greek yogurt or skyr, fresh mixed berries, chopped nuts and

seeds, honey or maple syrup (if using), and whole-grain muesli or granola (if desired).

2. Add Yogurt Base: Start by placing a portion of Greek yogurt or skyr at the bottom of a bowl. The amount can vary based on your preference.

3. Add Berries: Add a generous serving of fresh mixed berries on top of the yogurt. You can mix and match various berries for a burst of color and flavor.

4. Sprinkle Nuts and Seeds: Sprinkle a variety of chopped nuts and seeds over the berries and yogurt. This adds a satisfying crunch and provides healthy fats and additional nutrients.

5. Drizzle with Honey or Maple Syrup (Optional): If you desire extra sweetness, you can drizzle a small amount of honey or maple syrup over the top of the breakfast bowl. Use sweeteners sparingly to align with Scandi Sense Diet principles.

6. Add Whole-Grain Muesli or Granola (Optional): If you'd like to include whole-grain muesli or granola for added texture and fiber, you can do so at this stage.

7. Taste and Adjust: Taste the breakfast bowl and adjust the sweetness and texture by adding more toppings or drizzle if desired.

8. Serve: Your Scandi Sense Breakfast Bowl is ready to be served. Enjoy it as a healthy and delicious way to kick-start your day.

The preparation time for a Scandi Sense Breakfast Bowl is minimal and should take approximately 5-10 minutes.

Lunch: Scandi Sense Salad

Ingredients:

- A base of mixed greens (e.g., spinach, lettuce, arugula)
- Lean protein (e.g., grilled chicken, tofu, smoked salmon)
- Sliced cucumbers
- Cherry tomatoes
- Sliced bell peppers
- A simple dressing (olive oil and balsamic vinegar)
- Whole-grain rye crackers or bread (optional)

Instructions:

1. Gather your Ingredients: Collect the mixed greens, lean protein, cucumbers, cherry

tomatoes, bell peppers, and dressing. Additionally, you can include whole-grain rye crackers or bread if desired.

2. Prepare the Greens: Wash and dry the mixed greens, then arrange them on a serving plate or in a salad bowl.

3. Add Lean Protein: Place a generous portion (about 100g) of lean protein (grilled chicken, tofu, and smoked salmon) on top of the mixed greens. This serves as the protein source for your salad.

4. Layer with Vegetables: Add sliced cucumbers, cherry tomatoes, and sliced bell peppers on top of the protein. Feel free to use other vegetables of your choice for added variety and freshness.

5. Dress the Salad: Drizzle the salad with a simple dressing made from olive oil and balsamic vinegar. You can adjust the dressing quantity to suit your preference.

6. Add Whole-Grain Rye Crackers or Bread (Optional): If you'd like to add whole-grain rye crackers or bread to your salad, you can serve them on the side.

7. Toss or Serve: If you prefer, you can gently toss the salad to mix the ingredients. Alternatively, serve it as a composed salad with distinct layers.

8. Serve: Your Scandi Sense Salad is ready to be served. Enjoy it as a healthy and refreshing meal.

The preparation time for a Scandi Sense Salad is quick and should take approximately 10-15 minutes, depending on how long it takes to wash and chop the ingredients and assemble the salad.

Dinner: Scandi Sense Lentil and Vegetable Stew

Ingredients:

- Dry green or brown lentils
- Chopped vegetables (e.g., carrots, celery, onions)
- Olive oil
- Minced garlic
- Low-sodium vegetable broth
- Seasonings (e.g., thyme, bay leaves, salt, and pepper)
- Chopped fresh herbs (e.g., parsley)
- Optional protein (e.g., diced chicken or tofu)

Instructions:

1. Gather your Ingredients: Collect dry green or brown lentils, chopped vegetables, olive oil, minced garlic, low-sodium vegetable broth,

seasonings, chopped fresh herbs, and any optional protein (chicken or tofu).

2. Rinse the Lentils: Rinse the dry lentils in cold water and set them aside.

3. Sauté Vegetables: In a large pot or Dutch oven, heat a bit of olive oil over medium heat. Sauté the chopped vegetables (carrots, celery, onions) until they begin to soften and become fragrant.

4. Add Minced Garlic: Add minced garlic to the sautéed vegetables and cook for about a minute, or until fragrant.

5. Add Lentils and Broth: Add the rinsed lentils and low-sodium vegetable broth to the pot. The amount of broth can vary depending on the desired thickness of your stew.

6. Season the Stew: Season the stew with your choice of seasonings, such as thyme, bay leaves, salt, and pepper. Stir to combine.

7. Cook the Lentils: Bring the stew to a gentle simmer and cook for about 20-30 minutes, or until the lentils and vegetables are tender. The cooking time may vary based on the type and age of the lentils.

8. Add Fresh Herbs: In the final minutes of cooking, stir in chopped fresh herbs like parsley to add a burst of flavor and freshness.

9. Cook Optional Protein (if using): If you're including diced chicken or tofu, add them to the stew and simmer until they are cooked through.

10. Taste and Adjust: Taste the stew and adjust the seasoning if needed by adding more herbs, salt, or pepper.

11. Serve: Your Scandi Sense Lentil and Vegetable Stew is ready to be served. Ladle it into bowls and enjoy a hearty and balanced meal.

The preparation and cooking time for a Scandi Sense Lentil and Vegetable Stew typically takes around 40-50 minutes.

Day 7:

Breakfast: Scandi Sense Fruit and Nut Plate

Ingredients:

- Assorted fresh fruits (e.g., apples, pears, grapes, berries)
- A selection of nuts (e.g., almonds, walnuts, cashews)

- Optional cheese or yogurt

- A drizzle of honey (optional)

Instructions:

1. Gather Your Ingredients: Collect assorted fresh fruits, a selection of nuts, optional cheese or yogurt, and a small amount of honey (if using).

2. Prepare Fruits: Wash, peel (if desired), and slice the fresh fruits. Arrange them on a serving plate.

3. Add Nuts: Place a variety of nuts (e.g., almonds, walnuts, cashews) on the plate alongside the fresh fruits. Nuts add a satisfying crunch and healthy fats to the plate.

4. Include Cheese or Yogurt (Optional): If you'd like to add a protein component to your plate, you can include cheese or a small serving of yogurt.

5. Drizzle with Honey (Optional): For a touch of sweetness, drizzle a small amount of honey over the fruits, nuts, or cheese. Use honey sparingly to align with Scandi Sense Diet principles.

6. Taste and Adjust: Taste your Fruit and Nut Plate and adjust the sweetness or texture by adding more honey or other toppings if desired.

7. Serve: Your Scandi Sense Fruit and Nut Plate is ready to be served. Enjoy it as a nutritious and satisfying snack or light meal.

The preparation time for a Scandi Sense Fruit and Nut Plate is minimal, typically taking around 10-15 minutes.

Lunch: Scandi Sense Quinoa Salad

Ingredients:

- Quinoa
- Chopped vegetables (e.g., bell peppers, cucumbers, cherry tomatoes)
- Fresh herbs (e.g., parsley, mint)
- Olive oil and lemon juice for dressing
- Optional protein (e.g., grilled chicken, tofu, or chickpeas)
- Feta cheese (optional)
- Salt and pepper to taste

Instructions:

1. Gather Your Ingredients: Collect quinoa, chopped vegetables, fresh herbs, olive oil, lemon juice, optional protein (if using), and feta cheese (if desired).

2. Cook the Quinoa: Rinse the quinoa in cold water, then cook it according to the package instructions. Typically, the quinoa is simmered in water or broth for 15-20 minutes until it's fluffy and the liquid is absorbed. Once cooked, let it cool to room temperature.

3. Prepare the Vegetables: While the quinoa is cooking and cooling, chop the vegetables (bell peppers, cucumbers, cherry tomatoes) and fresh herbs (parsley, mint).

4. Make the Dressing: In a small bowl, whisk together olive oil and lemon juice to create a simple dressing. You can adjust the proportions to taste.

5. Add Vegetables and Herbs: In a large bowl, combine the cooked and cooled quinoa with the chopped vegetables and fresh herbs.

6. Drizzle with Dressing: Drizzle the dressing over the quinoa salad and toss everything together. Ensure that the salad is well coated with the dressing.

7. Add Optional Protein: If you're including grilled chicken, tofu, or chickpeas for added protein, mix them into the salad at this stage.

8. Season and Add Feta Cheese (Optional): Season the salad with salt and pepper to taste. If you like, you can crumble feta cheese over the top for added creaminess and flavor.

9. Taste and Adjust: Taste the quinoa salad and adjust the seasoning or dressing if needed.

10. Serve: Your Scandi Sense Quinoa Salad is ready to be served. Enjoy it as a balanced and satisfying meal.

The preparation time for a Scandi Sense Quinoa Salad typically takes around 30-40 minutes.

Dinner: Scandi Sense Beef Stir-fry

Ingredients:

- Lean beef (e.g., sirloin or flank steak) thinly sliced
- Assorted vegetables (e.g., bell peppers, broccoli, carrots, snap peas)
- Olive oil or cooking oil of your choice
- Minced garlic and ginger
- Low-sodium soy sauce or a light stir-fry sauce
- Whole grains (e.g., quinoa or brown rice)

Instructions:

1. Gather your Ingredients: Collect lean beef, assorted vegetables, olive oil or cooking oil, minced garlic, minced ginger, low-sodium soy sauce or stir-fry sauce, and whole grains.

2. Prepare the Beef: Slice the lean beef into thin strips. You can also marinate the beef with a bit of soy sauce and minced garlic for added flavor.

3. Cut the Vegetables: Chop the assorted vegetables into uniform, bite-sized pieces.

4. Heat the Pan: Heat a large skillet or wok over medium-high heat. Add a small amount of olive oil or cooking oil.

5. Sauté Garlic and Ginger: Add minced garlic and ginger to the hot skillet and stir-fry for about a minute until fragrant.

6. Stir-Fry Beef: Add the sliced beef to the skillet and stir-fry until its no longer pink. This should take a few minutes. Remove the cooked beef from the skillet and set it aside.

7. Sauté Vegetables: In the same skillet, add a bit more oil if needed. Stir-fry the chopped vegetables until they start to become tender yet still crisp.

8. Combine Beef and Vegetables: Return the cooked beef to the skillet with the sautéed vegetables. Toss everything together.

9. Add Sauce: Drizzle low-sodium soy sauce or your preferred stir-fry sauce over the beef and vegetable mixture. Toss to coat everything evenly and cook for a few more minutes.

10. Serve Over Whole Grains: Place a serving of cooked whole grains (quinoa or brown rice) on a plate or in a bowl. Top the grains with the beef and vegetable stir-fry.

11. Taste and Adjust: Taste the stir-fry and adjust the seasoning or sauce if needed.

12. Serve: Your Scandi Sense Beef Stir-Fry is ready to be served. Enjoy it as a balanced and flavorful meal.

The preparation and cooking time for a Scandi Sense Beef Stir-Fry typically takes around 20-30 minutes.

Preparation Tips

- Based on your weekly menu, make a grocery list and plan your meals in advance.

- To make cooking throughout the week easier, prepare certain things in advance. Examples of this include washing and cutting vegetables and marinating meats.

- To keep fruits and vegetables fresh throughout the week, store them appropriately.

- When preparing foods that may be used in many meals, such as grains or proteins, batch cooking is recommended.

- To reduce food waste, repurpose leftover components from one meal in another.

- Keep an eye on portion sizes and serve food in accordance with the proportion and balance principles of Scandi Sense.

Chapter 6

Weight Management with Scandi Sense

A key component of the Scandi Sense Diet, which places an emphasis on portion control and conscious, balanced eating, is weight management. This chapter will discuss the fundamentals of the Scandi Sense method to reaching and maintaining a healthy weight.

Understanding Healthy Weight: The goal of the Scandi Sense Diet is to help people reach and maintain a healthy weight that suits their unique body type, height, and general health. A practical and sustainable approach to weight control is prioritized above fad diets or unattainable body goals.

Balanced Nutrition: Balanced diet is one of the main methods for managing weight using Scandi Sense. This entails eating a range of meals high in nutrients in sensible serving sizes. With sections for veggies, proteins, carbs, and healthy fats, the Scandi Sense Plate acts as a visual aid for preparing meals that are well-balanced. This method guarantees that your body gets the vital nutrients it needs to perform at its best.

Portion Control: Another crucial component of using Scandi Sense for weight loss is portion control. You may efficiently control your calorie intake and avoid overeating by paying attention to portion sizes and according to the Scandi Sense Plate's guidelines. This may allow you to eat tasty, filling meals and maintain or even reach a healthy weight.

Energy Efficiency: The Scandi Sense Diet encourages long-term, sustainable weight control. Instead than depending on severe calorie restriction or deprivation, it helps people to have a healthy, fulfilling relationship with food. If necessary, this may result in long-term maintenance of a healthy weight and sustained weight decrease.

Activities Physical: The Scandi Sense Diet acknowledges the value of physical exercise for both weight control and general health, even if it's main emphasis is on eating behaviors. Including frequent exercise in your regimen may aid in weight reduction and help you keep it off.

Personalized Method: The Scandi Sense Diet recognizes that maintaining a healthy weight is a very personal endeavor. It doesn't enforce strict guidelines or universally applicable solutions. Rather, it empowers people to modify the guidelines according to their particular requirements and inclinations, encouraging a feeling of responsibility and independence in managing their weight.

Chapter 7

Enhanced Nutrition and Wellness

Nutrient-Rich Scandinavian Foods

The Scandi Sense Diet's emphasis on balance, diversity, and proportion is reflected in the many nutrient-rich foods found in Scandinavian cuisine. Some nutrient-dense Scandinavian cuisine are as follows:

1. Saturated Fish: Omega-3 fatty acids are abundant in fish such as salmon, mackerel, herring, and trout and are good for the heart and brain. They are also fantastic providers of top-notch protein.

2. Fruit: Cloudberries, blueberries, and lingonberries are among the many types of wild berries that are abundant in Scandinavian nations. These berries are a great source of fiber, vitamins, and antioxidants that promote general health and wellbeing.

3. Complete Grains: A mainstay of Scandinavian diets include barley, rye, and oats. These whole grains are a wonderful source of important vitamins, minerals, and dietary fiber. They are often added to porridge, bread, and other foods.

4. Vegetable Roots: In Scandinavian cooking, root vegetables including parsnips, turnips, and carrots are often employed. They are abundant in nutrients, vitamins, and fiber. For a nutrient-dense side dish, try roasted or mashed root veggies.

5. Lean Proteins: Scandinavian cuisine often features lean protein sources including tofu, lean meats, and fowl. They provide vital amino acids needed for healthy muscles and general wellbeing.

6. Milk-Based Goods: Milk, cheese, yogurt, and other dairy products are consumed by Scandinavians. For digestive health, they provide probiotics, calcium, and protein. For a healthy alternative, go for low-fat or fat-free selections.

7. Cruciferous vegetables: In Scandinavian cuisine, cabbage, broccoli, and cauliflower are often utilized vegetables. These veggies are great options for balanced meals since they're high in vitamins, fiber, and antioxidants.

8. Spices & Herbs from the North: Dill, cardamom, and cinnamon are just a few of the herbs and spices used in Scandinavian cooking. These spices enhance taste and may provide digestive

assistance and antioxidant support, among other health advantages.

9. Seeds and Nuts: Nuts like almonds and seeds like flaxseeds, which provide good fats, protein, and fiber, are often included in Scandinavian dishes. They work well as garnishes for salads and breakfast foods.

10. Fermented Foods: Scandinavian diets often include fermented foods such as kefir, pickled herring, and sauerkraut. Probiotics, which promote intestinal health and general wellbeing, are abundant in these foods.

11. Chocolate Dark: Antioxidant-rich dark chocolate is a popular treat in Scandinavia. Though dark chocolate may be a component of a nutrient-rich treat, moderation is crucial.

12. Canola Oil: Scandinavians often use canola oil for cooking since it is low in saturated fats and hence heart-healthy.

Benefits for Heart Health

Because of its focus on well-balanced, nutrient-rich, and portion-controlled meals, the Scandi Sense Diet may have several positive effects on heart health. Several heart-healthy advantages are linked to this eating strategy:

1. Lower Chance of Cardiovascular Conditions: The Scandi Sense Diet advocates for a diet high in veggies, healthy fats, lean meats, and whole grains. Eating these meals is linked to a lower risk of cardiovascular conditions, such as stroke and heart disease.

2. Omega-3 Fatty Acids: Omega-3 fatty acids may be found in abundance when fatty fish like herring, mackerel, and salmon are included. Studies have shown the anti-inflammatory, heart-healthy, and heart-risk-lowering effects of these important fats.

3. High-quality Protein: An essential component of the Scandi Sense Diet is lean proteins, including those found in chicken and lean meats. Protein maintains general health, including heart function, and is necessary for the health of muscles.

4. High-Fiber Foods: Dietary fiber is abundant in vegetables, berries, and whole grains. Fiber may assist improve heart health by lowering blood pressure, cholesterol, and blood pressure.

5. Handle Portion Size: Meal balance and portion management are the main focuses of the Scandi Sense Diet. Controlling portion sizes may help avoid overindulging, which is associated with increased risk of weight gain and heart disease.

6. Decreased Consumption of Sodium: Generally speaking, Scandinavian food utilizes less salt than a lot of other cuisines. Reducing salt consumption may aid in blood pressure management and lower the risk of heart disease and hypertension.

7. Few Refined Foods: The Scandi Sense Diet opposes the use of highly processed and packaged foods since they often have trans fats, excessive salt content, and added sugars, all of which are bad for the heart.

8. Beneficial Fats: Using heart-healthy fats, including those in nuts, seeds, and canola oil, may help lower the risk of heart disease. It is well recognized that these fats enhance cholesterol profiles and promote general heart health.

9. Rich in Antioxidants Berries: Antioxidants found in Scandinavian berries, such as lingonberries and blues, may help fight oxidative stress and

inflammation, two conditions that increase the risk of heart disease.

10. Ethical Consumption Practices: The Scandi Sense Diet encourages people to lessen their environmental footprint and supports sustainability. A sustainable diet that reduces resource misuse is good for the environment, which is good for human health and wellbeing.

Lowering the Risk of Chronic Diseases

Because it emphasizes portion management, conscious meal planning, and balanced, nutrient-rich eating, the Scandi Sense Diet may be a useful strategy for reducing the risk of chronic illnesses. This is how it may help lower the chance of developing chronic illnesses:

1. Heart Disease:
   - Well-Balanced Diet: A balanced consumption of nutrients, such as whole grains, vegetables, lean meats, and healthy fats, is encouraged by the diet. By lowering the chance of excessive blood pressure and dangerous cholesterol levels, this equilibrium promotes heart health.
   - Salivary Fats: Heart disease risk may be decreased and cholesterol profiles can be

improved by including fatty fish and heart-healthy fats from canola oil, nuts, and seeds.

- Control of Portion: People may prevent overeating, which is linked to weight gain and risk factors for heart disease, by adopting portion control.

2. Diabetes Type 2:

- Entire Grains: Whole grains are recommended because they are high in fiber. Consuming meals high in fiber may help control blood sugar levels and lower the chance of type 2 diabetes.

- Well-Composed Meals: Meals containing a balanced mix of carbs, proteins, and fats are encouraged by the Scandi Sense Diet, which may help control blood sugar levels.

- Control of Portion: Reducing portion sizes may help avoid consuming too many calories, which can help with weight control, which is crucial for managing and preventing diabetes.

3. Fatality:

- Control of Portion: Portion control is a key component of the Scandi Sense Diet, which helps people regulate their calorie intake, avoid overindulging, and maintain a healthy weight.

- Well-Balanced Diet: In order to help people feel full and reduce their tendency to overindulge, the diet encourages balanced meals that contain a range of nutrient-dense foods.

4. Elevated Blood Pressure: Hypertension:

- Decreased Salt: Less salt is used in Scandinavian cooking than in many other cuisines, which may assist reduce sodium consumption and minimize the risk of hypertension.

- Flora and Faunals: Consuming a diet high in fruits and vegetables supplies potassium, which may help offset the blood pressure-raising effects of salt.

- Control of Portion: Retaining proper portion sizes may help maintain blood pressure and weight by preventing overindulgence in calories.

5. Intestinal Conditions:

- Foods High in Fiber: High-fiber foods including whole grains, berries, and veggies are part of the diet. By encouraging regular bowel movements and lowering the risk of ailments like constipation and diverticular disease, fiber promotes digestive health.

- Probiotics: Probiotics included in fermented foods like kefir and sauerkraut help maintain a healthy gut microbiota and lower the risk of digestive problems.

6. Specific Cancers:

- Antioxidants: Packed in antioxidants, Scandinavian berries may lower the risk of several malignancies and fight oxidative stress.

- Complete Foods: Eating a diet high in whole, minimally processed foods lowers exposure to preservatives and additives, which may be detrimental and are linked to an increased risk of some malignancies.

7. Well-being of Mind:

- Conscious Consumption: By encouraging a better connection with food and minimizing emotional eating, mindful eating may improve mental health.

- Nutrition in Balance: The foundation of good general health, including mental health, is a well-rounded diet rich in necessary nutrients.

8. Ecological Viability:

- Scientific Health: The Scandi Sense Diet's emphasis on sustainable eating methods lessens the environmental effect of dietary decisions, improving long-term health by protecting the planet's health.

Chapter 8

Scandi Sense for the Whole Family

The whole family's health and wellbeing may be improved by modifying and implementing the Scandi Sense Diet. This chapter looks at how all family members, regardless of age, may adopt the values of balance, diversity, and proportion to support a healthy lifestyle.

Building Healthy Eating Habits in Children

One of the most important aspects of promoting family wellbeing in general is teaching children proper eating habits. Early exposure to a balanced diet helps youngsters develop a lifetime fondness for wholesome food. It's possible to modify the Scandi Sense Diet's portion management and balanced meal strategies to make recipes that the whole family will like.

Planning and Preparing Family Meals

It may be a fulfilling experience to plan and prepare meals for the family using the Scandi Sense Diet's tenets. The following are some tactics:

1. Diversity of Meals: To make sure that family members get the vital nutrients they need, plan a

variety of meals that contain lean meats, whole grains, veggies, and healthy fats.

2. Portion Control: Adjust serving sizes to suit individual family members' requirements. Children should have portions that are suitable for their age, but adults should be free to modify according to their own dietary needs.

3. Including Children: Involve kids in meal preparation and decision-making. This aids in their feeling of empowerment and comprehension of a healthy diet.

4. Sensitive Plate Scandi: It is simpler to adhere to the diet's tenets when meals are prepared for the whole family using the Scandi Sense Plate as a visual guide.

Mindful Eating for All Ages

All members of the family may benefit from the mindful eating practice. Family members may identify their hunger and fullness signals, enjoy meals more completely, and lower their chance of overeating by paying attention to the eating experience. This habit may be a useful one for kids to avoid emotional eating and foster a healthy connection with food.

Personalization and Adaptability

The adaptability of the Scandi Sense Diet is one of its advantages. It may be altered to suit dietary restrictions, ethnic backgrounds, and personal tastes. Families benefit from this flexibility since it enables them to make meals that satisfy their needs and preferences while adhering to the diet's guidelines.

Healthy Eating at Every Stage of Life

Everyone may benefit from the Scandi Sense Diet, regardless of age, from small children to the elderly. It is a flexible strategy that satisfies the nutritional requirements of every member of the family because of its emphasis on nutrient-rich meals, portion management, and balance.

Family Wellness beyond Food

Holistic family wellbeing is also promoted by the Scandi Sense Diet. Although diet plays a crucial role, it also acknowledges the significance of physical exercise, mental health, and leading a balanced lifestyle. To promote general health and connectedness, family members might partake in activities like physical activity, outdoor excursions, and leisurely meals together.

Chapter 9

Dining Out and Social Scenarios

By applying the balance, variety, and proportion principles of the Scandi Sense Diet to social situations and eating out, people may follow their nutritional objectives and yet enjoy social gatherings without jeopardizing their health and wellbeing.

Responsibly Eating Out

Maintaining a portion-controlled and well-balanced diet might be difficult while dining out. However, people may choose better options if they use thoughtful strategies:

1. Exploration of Menu: When eating out, spend some time perusing the menu. Seek for recipes that follow the guidelines of the Scandi Sense Diet, such as those that include plenty of veggies, healthy grains, and lean meats.

2. Adjustment: Please feel free to modify your purchase. To better align the meals with your dietary needs and tastes, ask that they be modified. For example, request dressing on the side or choose steamed rather than fried food.

3. Portion Awareness: Pay attention to the serving sizes at dining establishments. If you want to

reserve half of your dinner for later, ask for a to-go box or think about splitting an entrée with a dining partner.

4. Mindful Eating: Even while dining out, use mindful eating practices. Enjoy every mouthful, converse with others, and pay attention to your body's signals of hunger and fullness.

Social Scenarios and Celebrations

Numerous mouthwatering meals are often served at social events and festivities. The Scandi Sense Diet's tenets may be used in the following situations:

1. Setting Up: Have a modest, well-balanced supper or snack before heading out to avoid becoming too hungry. When presented with a variety of alternatives, this may assist you in making more deliberate decisions.

2. Control: In moderation, indulge in sweets and delights. Enjoy excellent foods in moderation rather than in excess.

3. Suggested Beverages: To keep hydrated and save calories overall, choose water or other low-calorie drinks, especially in places where sugar-filled or alcoholic beverages are served often.

4. Social Support: Tell your loved ones about your dietary objectives. They may provide empathy and support, which makes it simpler to handle social situations without feeling compelled to stray from your chosen course.

Travel and On-the-Go Eating

Regular meal times may be disturbed by travel and hectic schedules, but the Scandi Sense Diet can still be adhered to:

1. Snack Packing: Make healthy snacks like whole-grain crackers, fresh fruit, and almonds for when you're on the go or have a hectic day. This guarantees that you will always have wholesome selections on hand.

2. Regional Food: When you travel, try local cuisines that follow the guidelines of the plan. This will let you enjoy new foods while still eating a balanced diet.

3. Meal Planning: Try to schedule meals in advance by calling ahead at restaurants or looking out neighborhood eateries that provide wholesome fare.

Flexibility and Adaptability: The Scandi Sense Diet is adaptable to various situations. It encourages individuals to be flexible while adhering to the principles of balance, variety, and proportion. While there may be occasional indulgences in social scenarios or while dining out, these can be balanced by making mindful choices and following the diet's principles in the majority of meals.

Chapter 10

Eco-Friendly Eating

A cornerstone of the Scandi Sense Diet is eco-friendly eating, often known as sustainable eating. This chapter examines how this eating strategy promotes the health of people and the environment by adhering to sustainability and environmental responsibility principles.

The Effects of Food Choices on the Environment: The Scandi Sense Diet recognizes that dietary decisions people make have a big influence on the environment. Food production, distribution, and disposal have the potential to worsen resource depletion, habitat loss, and greenhouse gas emissions. People may help the planet's health and lessen their environmental impact by adopting eco-friendly eating habits.

Seasonal and Local Produce: A fundamental principle of environmentally conscious eating is prioritizing seasonal and locally grown vegetables. People following the Scandi Sense Diet are encouraged to include fruits, vegetables, and other foods that are produced locally and in season. They help local farmers and lessen the carbon emissions brought on by the long-distance delivery of food by doing this.

Minimizing Food Waste: Reducing food waste is essential to eating sustainably. Meal planning and portion management are encouraged by the Scandi Sense Diet, which may assist people in minimizing food waste. People may reduce the quantity of food that ends up in landfills by just buying and cooking what they need.

Options for Sustainable Protein: The diet promotes the intake of plant-based proteins, reduces the amount of meat from non-sustainable sources, and favors fatty fish from well-managed fisheries. Selecting sustainable protein sources helps lessen the negative environmental effects of raising animals and save marine habitats.

Decreased Intake of Processed Foods: Because more processed foods need more energy and resources to produce, they often have a larger environmental impact. The Scandi Sense Diet suggests that people should consume less packaged and processed meals in favor of whole or minimally processed foods. This decision reduces the environmental effect of food processing, which is in line with sustainable eating.

Single-Use Plastics Used Minimally: Beyond only food choices, the diet encourages environmentally sustainable behavior. It encourages people to use less single-use plastics, such straws, throwaway containers, and plastic cutlery. By doing this, plastic waste is reduced along with its harmful consequences on the environment.

Maintaining Food Systems Sustainable: Sustainable food systems are supported by eco-friendly eating practices. The Marine Stewardship Council, Fair Trade, and organic certificates are just a few examples of the certifications that those following the Scandi Sense Diet are encouraged to look for on food goods.

Health of the Individual and the Environment: Eating sustainably has a direct impact on one's health. Whole foods high in nutrients that follow the guidelines of the Scandi Sense Diet benefit people's health and wellbeing while also benefiting the environment. In keeping with the diet's dedication to balance and proportion, a diet high in fruits, vegetables, whole grains, and lean proteins may lower the risk of chronic illnesses and promote long-term health.

Chapter 11

The Scandi Sense Lifestyle

The Scandi Sense Diet is a comprehensive lifestyle strategy that emphasizes balance, awareness, and overall well-being. It goes beyond simple dietary choices. This chapter explores the wider facets of the Scandi Sense way of living and how it contributes to a happier, healthier existence.

Creative Existence: A fundamental component of the Scandi Sense way of living is mindfulness. It entails living in the present moment, whether you're having a meal, interacting with others, or enjoying a leisurely stroll. Being mindful may improve one's ability to appreciate life's little joys and assist in improving stress and mood management.

Link between Nature and the Outdoors: Scandinavian nations are well known for their closeness to the natural world. Whether it's taking a leisurely walk through the woods, hiking in the mountains, or just taking in the fresh air, the Scandi Sense lifestyle promotes spending time outside. A connection to nature has been linked to lowered stress levels and enhanced mental health.

Social and Family Ties: In order to develop stronger bonds and emotional wellbeing, the Scandi Sense Diet encourages family dinners and get-togethers. Spending time with loved ones around the table promotes candid discussion, deepens relationships, and improves life quality.

Workout and Physical Activity: Although the diet mostly focuses on food selections, the Scandi Sense way of life acknowledges the need of consistent exercise. Including exercise in everyday activities may boost mental health, increase physical fitness, and promote general wellbeing.

Equitable Integration of Work and Life: For general wellbeing, work and personal life must be balanced. People that follow the Scandi Sense lifestyle are encouraged to set boundaries, give self-care first priority, and have a good work-life balance. This strategy may lessen stress and keep burnout at bay.

Earth-friendly Living: One aspect of sustainability in the Scandi Sense lifestyle is eco-friendly dining. People are urged to adopt sustainable practices in various spheres of their lives, such cutting down on waste, preserving resources, and choosing products that don't harm the environment.

Simple Pleasures Enjoyed: The Scandi Sense way of living emphasizes appreciating the little things in life. Savoring these moments, whether it's a quiet moment of introspection, a cup of tea with a friend, or a cozy afternoon by the fireplace, leads to a deeper feeling of satisfaction and happiness.

Awareness of Seasons: The way of life recognizes the cyclical nature of existence and corresponds with the seasons. Celebrate and enjoy the changing of the seasons via cuisine, outdoor activities, and cultural customs.

Cultural and Gastronomic Discovery: The Scandi Sense way of life promotes learning about many cultures and cuisines. People's enjoyment of the culinary world may be further enhanced by expanding their horizons, which allows them to taste new sensations and appreciate the richness of worldwide customs.

Minimalism and Simplicity: A cornerstone of the Scandi Sense way of life is simplicity. It highlights the elegance of minimalism, in which function and quality are more important than extravagance. Clarity and less stress might result from simplifying one's life.

Conclusion

Embrace a Healthier, Balanced, and Fulfilling Life with Scandi Sense

You have entered a world where food becomes nutrition, balance becomes a guiding principle, and awareness becomes a way of life as you explore the Scandi Sense Diet. This nutritional strategy, which has its roots in the core of Scandinavian customs, provides a comprehensive overhaul of your lifestyle in addition to a way to become a healthier version of yourself.

You now know that the Scandi Sense Diet is about enjoying life to the fullest that is, it's about cooking with joy, eating with pleasure, and mastering the skill of savoring every meal. It all comes down to finding the ideal balance between enjoyment and nutrition, so that you may eat your favorite foods guilt-free and yet experience health benefits.

You have now experienced the fundamental ideas of Scandi Sense:

1. Balance: The skill of proportion, wherein the proteins, veggies, carbs, and good fats on your plate are perfectly balanced. It's about embracing diversity and moderation, not about deprivation.

2. Mindfulness: Eating mindfully, appreciating each bite, and paying attention to your body's signals when eating. It's about regaining the joy of eating and reestablishing a connection with food.

3. Eco-Friendly Eating: A dedication to sustainability in which the foods you eat are in line with your moral principles and benefit the environment. It has to do with taking care of the Earth as well as oneself.

4. Wellness beyond Food: Acknowledging that living a healthy lifestyle goes beyond what you eat. It includes being active, feeling good about oneself, spending time with family, and having a close relationship with the natural world.

You've accepted not only the Scandi Sense Diet but a lifestyle that extends beyond the kitchen. You'll be able to connect with the world around you, enjoy the cyclical beauty of the seasons, and find delight in the little things in life.

You have unlocked a wealth of gastronomic pleasures, health-conscious options, and a revitalized sense of global connectedness by learning about the Scandi Sense Diet. It is a voyage of self-love, self-discovery, and self-care.

As you go along this route, keep in mind that the Scandi Sense Diet is neither a short-term fix nor a rigid routine. This is a way of life that is here to stay and may greatly improve your quality of life.

So, my dear reader, enjoy every meal, treasure every moment, and take care of your health as you set off on your Scandi Sense trip. Allow the Scandi Sense Diet to lead you to a life of increased contentment, pleasure, and wellbeing as you experience the delight of balanced living. It's time to savor each morsel and rediscover the allure of living a Scandi Sense lifestyle.

9 798887 044039